How not to die early in life

By John P Hale

Table of Contents

Chapter 1: Nutrition Matters

- Basics of Good Nutrition

- Foods to Embrace and Foods to Avoid

- Meal Planning for a Healthy Life

- The Importance of Hydration

Chapter 2: Exercise: The Essence of Life

- Benefits of Regular Physical Activity

- Types of Exercises for Different Age Groups

- Creating a Sustainable Workout Routine

- The Role of Movement in Mental Health

Chapter 3: Mental Health and Well-being

- Understanding Stress and Its Effects on the Body

- Techniques for Managing Stress (Meditation, Mindfulness, Therapy)

- Importance of Social Connections and Support Systems

- Recognizing the Signs of Mental Health Issues

Chapter 4: Prevention is Key

- Routine Check-ups and Screenings

- Vaccinations and Their Importance

- Understanding Family Medical History

- Self-examination and Early Detection (e.g., for cancer)

Chapter 5: Safety First

- Home Safety Tips (Fire, Falls, Carbon Monoxide)

- Road Safety and Driving Precautions

- Personal Safety and Awareness

- Emergency Preparedness (First Aid, Natural Disasters)

Chapter 6: Managing Risks

- Understanding and Managing Chronic Conditions

- Avoiding harmful substances (tobacco, excessive alcohol, drugs)

- Cybersecurity and Mental Well-being in a Digital Age

Chapter 7: Lifestyle Changes for Longevity

- The Importance of Sleep and Rest

- Reducing Toxic Relationships

- Setting Goals for a Fulfilling Life

- Engaging in Hobbies and Lifelong Learning

Chapter 8: Case Studies and Real-Life Examples

- Stories from Individuals Who Made Positive Changes

- Lessons Learned from Tragedies and Near-Deaths

- Interviews with Health Professionals

Chapter 1: Nutrition Matters

Introduction to Nutrition

Nutrition is the cornerstone of a healthy life. It encompasses the processes by which our bodies take in and utilize food, impacting everything from physical health to mental well-being. In this chapter, we'll explore the essentials of good nutrition, examine the foods that nourish our bodies, and learn how to create a sustainable and enjoyable eating plan.

The Basics of Good Nutrition

Nutrition involves several key components:

1. **Macronutrients**: These are the nutrients our bodies need in larger amounts.

   - **Carbohydrates**: The body's primary energy source. Focus on whole grains, fruits, and vegetables.

   - **Proteins**: Essential for building and repairing tissues. Include lean meats, fish, legumes, and dairy.

   - **Fats**: Necessary for hormone production and cell health. Opt for healthy fats from sources like avocados, nuts, and olive oil.

2. **Micronutrients**: These are vitamins and minerals required in smaller amounts but are vital for overall health.

   - **Vitamins**: Organic compounds that support metabolic processes. Important examples include Vitamin C (found in citrus fruits) and Vitamin D (from sunlight and fortified foods).

   - **Minerals**: Inorganic elements like iron, calcium, and magnesium that play crucial roles in bodily functions.

3. **Fiber**: A type of carbohydrate that aids digestion and promotes a feeling of fullness. Sources include whole grains, fruits, vegetables, and legumes.

Foods to Embrace and Foods to Avoid

Foods to Embrace:

- **Fruits and Vegetables**: Aim for a rainbow of colors on your plate to ensure a diverse range of nutrients.

- **Whole Grains**: Brown rice, quinoa, oats, and whole grain bread are better alternatives to refined grains.

- **Lean Proteins**: Prioritize fish, poultry, beans, tofu, and nuts over red meats.

- **Healthy Fats**: Incorporate sources of omega-3 fatty acids, such as salmon, chia seeds, and walnuts.

Foods to Avoid:

- **Processed Foods**: Often high in sugars, unhealthy fats, and sodium. Examples include sugary snacks, fast food, and ready-to-eat meals.

- **Sugary Beverages**: Soft drinks and energy drinks can lead to excessive calorie intake and poor nutrition.

- **Excessive Salt**: High sodium intake is linked to hypertension and other health issues. Opt for herbs and spices for flavor instead of salt.

Meal Planning for a Healthy Life

Creating a meal plan can simplify shopping and cooking while ensuring a balanced diet. Here are a few tips:

1. **Plan Your Meals**: Take an hour each week to map out meals incorporating diverse food groups.

2. **Make a Shopping List**: Stick to whole foods and limit the purchase of processed snacks.

3. **Prep Ahead**: Batch cooking and preparing snacks in advance can save time and help you make healthier choices during busy days.

The Importance of Hydration

Water is essential for nearly every function in our bodies. It aids digestion, regulates temperature, and nourishes cells.

- Aim for about 8 cups (64 ounces) of water a day, but individual needs may vary based on activity level and climate.

- Limit consumption of sugary drinks and caffeinated beverages, which can lead to dehydration.

Conclusion

Nutrition plays an essential role in preventing illness, promoting physical fitness, and enhancing mental clarity. By adopting a balanced approach to eating and making informed choices about what we consume, we can significantly improve our quality of life. In the next chapter, we'll explore the importance of exercise and how it complements nutrition for a healthier lifestyle.

By understanding and applying these nutritional principles, you're taking a critical step toward ensuring you don't just live longer, but that you thrive in your everyday life.

Chapter 2: Exercise: The Essence of Life

Introduction to Exercise

In the pursuit of a healthy life, exercise is as vital as nutrition. It not only strengthens our bodies but also boosts our mental health and overall well-being. In this chapter, we'll discover the numerous benefits of regular physical activity, explore different types of exercises, and learn how to create a sustainable workout routine that fits into our lifestyles.

Benefits of Regular Physical Activity

Engaging in regular exercise provides a multitude of benefits that can enhance both physical and mental health:

1. **Improved Physical Health**: Regular exercise strengthens the heart, improves circulation, and enhances cardiovascular fitness. It also supports weight management and reduces the risk of chronic diseases such as diabetes, heart disease, and certain cancers.

2. **Enhanced Mental Health**: Physical activity is linked to improved mood and decreased symptoms of anxiety and depression. Exercise releases endorphins, often referred to as "feel-good" hormones, leading to a natural uplift in mood.

3. **Boosted Energy Levels**: Regular exercise improves muscle strength, endurance, and overall energy levels. As cardiovascular efficiency improves, daily tasks become easier and less tiring.

4. **Better Sleep**: Engaging in physical activity can help you fall asleep faster and deepen your sleep, thus combating insomnia and restlessness.

Types of Exercises for Different Age Groups

Exercise is not one-size-fits-all; different types can benefit individuals at various stages of life:

1. **Aerobic Exercise**: Activities like walking, running, swimming, and cycling elevate your heart rate and improve cardiovascular health. Aim for at least 150 minutes of moderate-intensity aerobic activity each week.

2. **Strength Training**: Lifting weights, resistance bands, or body-weight exercises (like push-ups and squats) build muscle and bone strength. Include strength training twice a week to gain its benefits.

3. **Flexibility and Balance**: Stretching, yoga, and tai chi help maintain flexibility and balance, reducing the risk of injuries, particularly as we age.

4. **High-Intensity Interval Training (HIIT)**: Alternating between short bursts of intense activity and lower-intensity recovery periods, HIIT workouts are efficient and effective for burning calories and improving fitness.

5. **Lifestyle Movement**: Incorporating more movement into daily life—like taking the stairs instead of the elevator, gardening, or playing with children—can enhance overall activity levels.

Creating a Sustainable Workout Routine

Establishing a workout routine that suits your schedule and preferences is crucial for long-term adherence. Here are some tips to create a sustainable plan:

1. **Set Realistic Goals**: Start small and gradually increase the intensity and duration of workouts. Setting achievable goals helps build confidence and motivation.

2. **Choose Activities You Enjoy**: If you dislike running, try dancing, cycling, or group classes. The more you enjoy the activity, the more likely you are to stick with it.

3. **Schedule Your Workouts**: Treat your exercise time like an important appointment. Schedule specific days and times to work out, making it a non-negotiable part of your routine.

4. **Mix It Up**: To prevent boredom and work different muscle groups, vary your activities. Alternating between cardio, strength, and flexibility exercises can also prevent overuse injuries.

5. **Incorporate Social Elements**: Join classes or workout groups to stay motivated, meet new people, and hold yourself accountable.

Overcoming Barriers to Exercise

Barriers such as time constraints, lack of motivation, or injury can hinder exercise habits. Here's how to overcome them:

- **Time Management**: Break workouts into shorter sessions (10-15 minutes) throughout the day if longer sessions feel daunting.

- **Find Motivation**: Track your progress, celebrate achievements, and remind yourself of the reasons you want to stay fit.

- **Start Slow**: If you're new to exercise or returning after a break, start with low-impact workouts and gradually increase intensity to avoid injury.

Conclusion

Exercise is truly the essence of life, providing significant benefits that go beyond just physical health. Regular physical activity enhances mental clarity, boosts mood, and fosters resilience against various health issues. By understanding the different types of exercise, creating a personalized routine, and overcoming barriers, you can incorporate physical activity into your life in a meaningful way.

In the next chapter, we'll dive into the critical connection between mental health and well-being, exploring how exercise and mental wellness go hand in hand. Remember, the journey to a healthier life is as much about movement as it is about nourishment, and every step counts.

Chapter 3: Mental Health and Well-being

Introduction to Mental Health

Mental health is a fundamental aspect of our overall well-being, influencing how we think, feel, and act. It encompasses our emotional, psychological, and social health and affects how we handle stress, relate to others, and make choices. This chapter will explore the significance of mental health, the impact of stress, effective coping techniques, and the importance of fostering strong social connections.

Understanding Stress and Its Effects

Stress is a natural response to life's challenges and can be both positive and negative. While short-term stress can motivate us to meet deadlines or face new experiences, chronic stress can lead to serious mental and physical health issues.

1. **Signs of Chronic Stress**:

   - Anxiety, irritability, or mood swings

   - Fatigue or sleep disturbances

   - Difficulty concentrating

   - Physical symptoms like headaches or stomach issues

2. **Long-Term Effects of Stress**:

   Chronic stress can contribute to various health problems, including heart disease, obesity, diabetes, depression, and anxiety disorders. Recognizing and managing stress is crucial for maintaining mental health.

Techniques for Managing Stress

Implementing healthy coping strategies can significantly mitigate the effects of stress:

1. **Mindfulness and Meditation**: Practicing mindfulness involves being present in the moment without judgment. Techniques like deep breathing, meditation, and yoga can help calm the mind and reduce stress.

2. **Physical Activity**: As discussed in the previous chapter, exercise is a powerful stress reliever. It releases endorphins, improves mood, and can serve as an outlet for frustration.

3. **Journaling**: Writing down thoughts and feelings can help gain clarity and perspective. It can also be a valuable tool for processing emotions and identifying patterns of stress.

4. **Limitance of Screen Time**: Reducing time spent on social media and electronic devices can lower anxiety and improve mental clarity.

5. **Professional Help**: Speaking with a mental health professional, such as a therapist or counselor, can provide strategies tailored to individual needs and situations.

Importance of Social Connections and Support Systems

Strong social connections are vital for emotional resilience and mental well-being:

1. **Building a Support Network**: Cultivating relationships with family, friends, or community groups can provide a safety net during tough times. Sharing experiences and feelings can foster a sense of belonging and decrease isolation.

2. **Engagement in Activities**: Participating in group activities, clubs, or volunteering can enhance social connections and improve mood.

3. **Open Communication**: Learning to express thoughts and emotions openly can strengthen relationships and provide relief from emotional burdens.

4. **Recognizing Toxic Relationships**: It's essential to acknowledge relationships that drain your energy or create negativity. Evaluating and, if necessary, distancing yourself from toxic influences can boost mental health.

Recognizing the Signs of Mental Health Issues

Awareness of mental health issues is crucial for early intervention. Some common signs include:

- Persistent sadness or hopelessness

- Withdrawal from social activities

- Changes in appetite or sleep patterns

- Substance abuse or risky behaviors

- Extreme mood swings or irrational behavior

If you or someone you know is experiencing these symptoms, reaching out for help is a critical step.

Conclusion

Mental health is just as important as physical health and deserves our attention and care. By understanding the impact of stress, implementing effective coping strategies, and fostering supportive relationships, we can cultivate resilience and enhance our overall well-being.

As we navigate through life, remember that seeking help and prioritizing mental health is a sign of strength. In the next chapter, we will focus on prevention strategies, emphasizing the importance of routine check-ups and self-care to maintain health and well-being. Together, we can create a holistic approach to living a vibrant, fulfilling life.

Chapter 4: Prevention is Key

Introduction to Preventive Health

Prevention is an essential pillar of maintaining overall health and well-being. While treating illnesses is important, preventing them from occurring in the first place is far more effective in ensuring a long, healthy life. This chapter will explore key prevention strategies, the importance of routine check-ups, vaccinations, understanding family medical history, and self-examinations for early detection.

Routine Check-ups and Screenings

Regular health check-ups help detect potential issues before they develop into more serious problems. Routine screenings are essential for people of all ages, as they can identify health risks early.

1. **Annual Health Check-ups**:

   - **Blood Pressure**: Monitoring blood pressure is vital to prevent cardiovascular diseases.

   - **Cholesterol Levels**: Regular cholesterol screenings can help assess the risk of heart disease.

   - **Blood Sugar**: Testing for diabetes can help identify pre-diabetes and allow for early intervention.

2. **Age-Appropriate Screenings**:

   - **Women**: Pap smears and mammograms are crucial for early detection of cervical and breast cancers.

   - **Men**: Prostate exams and testicular checks are vital for men's health.

   - **Both**: Colonoscopies are recommended starting at age 45 to screen for colorectal cancer.

3. **Discussion with Health Providers**: It's essential to communicate with your healthcare provider about personal and family medical history, which can influence the type and frequency of screenings needed.

Vaccinations and Their Importance

Vaccinations are one of the most effective ways to prevent infectious diseases. Staying current with vaccines protects not only individual health but also public health.

1. **Childhood Vaccinations**: Parents should ensure their children receive vaccinations according to recommended schedules to protect against diseases like measles, mumps, and rubella.

2. **Adult Vaccines**: Adults should keep up with vaccines such as the flu shot, tetanus booster, and, if eligible, the shingles and pneumonia vaccines. The COVID-19 vaccine has also become an essential part of preventive health.

3. **Travel Vaccinations**: If traveling to certain countries, additional vaccines may be required to protect against diseases endemic to those regions.

Understanding Family Medical History

Knowledge of family medical history can play a critical role in preventive health:

1. **Identify Risks**: Understanding genetic predispositions to conditions like heart disease, diabetes, or certain cancers can prompt earlier screenings and lifestyle changes.

2. **Stay Informed**: Discuss medical history with family members and keep a written record. Share this information with healthcare providers to tailor preventive measures.

3. **Genetic Testing**: For those with a significant family history of genetic conditions, consider discussing genetic testing options with healthcare professionals.

Self-Examination and Early Detection

Self-examinations are a proactive way to monitor your health and catch potential issues early on:

1. **Breast Self-Exam**: Women should perform monthly breast self-exams to notice any changes or lumps and report them to a healthcare provider.

2. **Testicular Self-Exam**: Men should regularly check for unusual lumps in the testicles, which could indicate health issues.

3. **Skin Checks**: Regularly examining your skin for new moles or changes in existing moles can assist in early detection of skin cancer.

4. **Oral Health**: Monitoring your mouth for any unusual sores or lesions can prompt timely dental check-ups.

Conclusion

Prevention is indeed key to a longer, healthier life. By actively engaging in routine check-ups, staying current with vaccinations, understanding family medical history, and conducting self-examinations, individuals can significantly reduce their risk of developing severe health issues.

In the next chapter, we will explore the critical aspects of safety—emphasizing home safety, road safety, and personal security. By following preventative practices in various areas of life, we can create a holistic approach to health and well-being, ensuring we thrive in all aspects of our lives. Taking initiative today can lead to a healthier tomorrow.

Chapter 5: Safety First

Introduction to Safety

Safety is a critical component of living a healthy and fulfilling life. By prioritizing safety, we can reduce accidents, prevent injuries, and create a secure environment for ourselves and those around us. This chapter will discuss various safety measures, including home safety tips, road safety practices, personal safety awareness, and emergency preparedness.

Home Safety Tips

Your home should be a sanctuary, but accidents can happen if safety measures are overlooked. Here are essential tips to enhance home safety:

1. **Fall Prevention**:

   - Remove tripping hazards, such as loose rugs, clutter, and electrical cords.

   - Install handrails on staircases and grab bars in bathrooms.

   - Ensure good lighting in hallways and on staircases.

2. **Fire Safety**:

   - Install smoke detectors on every level of your home and test them monthly.

   - Create and practice a fire escape plan with your family.

   - Keep a fire extinguisher in easily accessible locations, such as the kitchen and garage.

3. **Carbon Monoxide (CO) Detection**:

   - Install a CO detector near sleeping areas and ensure it is functioning properly.

  - Be mindful of potential CO sources, such as gas appliances, and get them inspected regularly.

4. **Childproofing**:

   - If you have young children, secure furniture to walls and store hazardous substances out of their reach.

   - Use safety gates, outlet covers, and cabinet locks for added protection.

5. **Emergency Contacts**:

   - Keep a list of emergency numbers (fire department, police, poison control) in a visible spot and ensure all family members are aware of them.

Road Safety and Driving Precautions

Whether you're a driver or a pedestrian, road safety is paramount to preventing accidents:

1. **Safe Driving Practices**:

   - Always wear a seatbelt and ensure all passengers do the same.

   - Avoid distractions, including texting or using your phone while driving.

   - Obey speed limits and traffic signs, and never drive under the influence of alcohol or drugs.

2. **Defensive Driving**:

   - Be aware of other drivers and anticipate potential hazards.

  - Maintain a safe following distance and adjust speed according to road conditions.

3. **Pedestrian Safety**:

  - Always use crosswalks and wait for the pedestrian signal before crossing streets.

  - Stay alert and avoid using electronic devices while walking near traffic.

4. **Bike Safety**:

  - Wear a helmet and reflective clothing when cycling to be visible to drivers.

  - Follow traffic rules and signals just as vehicles do.

Personal Safety and Awareness

Being aware of your surroundings and taking proactive measures can enhance personal safety:

1. **Situational Awareness**:

  - Pay attention to your environment, especially in unfamiliar areas or crowded spaces.

  - Trust your instincts; if something feels off, seek help or remove yourself from the situation.

2. **Self-Defense**:

  - Consider taking self-defense classes to build confidence and learn techniques for protecting yourself.

3. **Travel Safety**:

   - Keep your belongings secure and be mindful of pickpockets in crowded areas.

   - Share your travel itinerary with a trusted friend or family member.

4. **Emergency Preparedness**:

   - Create an emergency kit with essentials such as water, non-perishable food, a flashlight, batteries, and first-aid supplies.

   - Prepare for natural disasters by knowing evacuation routes and having a family communication plan in place.

Conclusion

Prioritizing safety is essential in every aspect of our lives. From creating a secure home environment to practicing road safety and being vigilant in personal safety, these measures can significantly reduce the risk of accidents and injuries.

In the next chapter, we will explore the importance of managing risks, including chronic conditions and avoiding harmful substances. By adopting a proactive mindset toward safety, we can enhance our quality of life and cultivate an environment that supports health and well-being. Remember, a little prevention today can contribute to a lifetime of safety and security.

Chapter 6: Managing Risks

Introduction to Risk Management

Managing risks is a vital component of maintaining a healthy and fulfilling life. By identifying potential risks and taking proactive steps to mitigate them, we can significantly reduce the likelihood of serious health issues and improve our overall quality of life. This chapter will delve into understanding and managing chronic conditions, avoiding harmful substances, and embracing a proactive approach to personal and public safety.

Understanding and Managing Chronic Conditions

Chronic conditions—such as diabetes, heart disease, obesity, and hypertension—affect millions of people worldwide. Effectively managing these conditions requires a multifaceted approach:

1. **Regular Monitoring**:

   - Keep track of essential health indicators related to your chronic condition, such as blood sugar levels for diabetes or blood pressure readings for hypertension.

   - Regular check-ups with a healthcare provider can help adjust treatment plans as needed.

2. **Medication Management**:

   - Take medications as prescribed, and discuss any side effects or concerns with your doctor.

   - Use pill organizers or mobile apps to maintain adherence to medication schedules.

3. **Lifestyle Modifications**:

   - Adopt a balanced diet rich in whole foods, fruits, vegetables, and lean proteins to support overall health.

- Incorporate regular physical activity tailored to your abilities and limitations. Exercise has been shown to improve outcomes for many chronic conditions.

4. **Education and Support**:

   - Educate yourself about your condition through reliable sources, and consider joining support groups to connect with others facing similar challenges.

   - Discuss nutrition, exercise, and mental health strategies with professionals who can provide personalized guidance.

Avoiding Harmful Substances

Substance use can significantly impact your health and exacerbate existing conditions. Here are key areas of focus for avoidance:

1. **Tobacco**:

   - Smoking poses severe risks to health, including lung cancer, heart disease, and respiratory issues. If you smoke, seek support for cessation; many resources are available, including counseling and medications.

2. **Excessive Alcohol Consumption**:

   - While moderate alcohol consumption may be acceptable for some, excessive drinking can lead to addiction, liver disease, and other health issues. Understand what constitutes moderate drinking and consider alternatives if you're at risk.

3. **Recreational Drugs**:

- Using illicit drugs can pose additional health risks and may interfere with medications and treatments for chronic conditions. Seek support if you or someone you know struggles with substance use.

4. **Unregulated Supplements**:

   - Be cautious with dietary supplements or herbal remedies that aren't regulated. They may interact with prescription medications or lead to unexpected side effects. Always discuss supplements with a healthcare professional.

Cybersecurity and Mental Well-being in a Digital Age

Managing risks extends beyond physical health to include mental health and cybersecurity in our increasingly digital world:

1. **Mental Well-being**:

   - Limit exposure to negative news and toxic social media interactions that can contribute to anxiety and depression. Curate your online environment to include positive influences and supportive communities.

   - Set boundaries on screen time, focusing on real-life interactions and activities that promote well-being.

2. **Cybersecurity Measures**:

   - Protect personal information by using strong, unique passwords for accounts and enabling two-factor authentication where available.

   - Be cautious with sharing personal information online and aware of phishing schemes or online scams.

3. **Data Exposure Awareness**:

   - Regularly review and update privacy settings on social media platforms, and be mindful of what is shared publicly.

Conclusion

Managing risks proactively is essential for ensuring a sound mind and a healthy body. By understanding and managing chronic conditions, avoiding harmful substances, and being mindful of digital well-being, you can create a supportive environment that encourages health and happiness.

In the final chapter, we will review the holistic approach to health and well-being, emphasizing the interconnectedness of nutrition, exercise, mental health, prevention, safety, and risk management. As we cultivate these practices, we pave the way for a vibrant and fulfilling life. Remember, the choices we make today lay the foundation for a healthier tomorrow.

Chapter 7: Lifestyle Changes for Longevity

Introduction to Longevity

Living a long and healthy life is not merely a matter of genetics; it's heavily influenced by the lifestyle choices we make every day. Implementing specific changes in our daily routines can promote longevity and enhance our overall quality of life. In this chapter, we will explore essential lifestyle changes, including the importance of sleep, stress reduction, building positive relationships, engaging in lifelong learning, and finding purpose in life.

The Importance of Sleep and Rest

Quality sleep is one of the cornerstones of good health and longevity. Lack of sleep can lead to numerous health issues, including obesity, heart disease, diabetes, and impaired cognitive function.

1. **Establish a Sleep Routine**:

   - Aim for 7-9 hours of sleep per night by going to bed and waking up at the same time each day.

   - Create a calming bedtime routine, such as reading or practicing relaxation techniques, to signal your body that it's time to wind down.

2. **Optimize Your Sleep Environment**:

   - Keep your bedroom dark, cool, and quiet. Consider blackout curtains, earplugs, or white-noise machines to enhance your sleep environment.

   - Limit exposure to screens and blue light in the evening as it can interfere with your sleep cycle.

3. **Prioritize Naps**:

   - If you're struggling to get enough rest at night, a short nap during the day can provide a boost in alertness and improve mood.

Reducing Stress and Adopting Mindfulness

Chronic stress is linked to numerous health risks, including heart disease and a weakened immune system. Finding effective ways to manage stress can improve both physical and mental health.

1. **Mindfulness and Meditation**:

- Regular mindfulness practices, such as meditation and deep-breathing exercises, can help calm the mind and reduce stress levels. Aim for a few minutes each day to practice being present.

2. **Limit Multitasking**:

   - Focus on one task at a time to reduce stress caused by feeling overwhelmed. Breaking tasks into manageable steps can make them feel less daunting.

3. **Engage in Hobbies**:

   - Engage in activities you enjoy regularly, whether reading, gardening, crafting, or playing a musical instrument. Hobbies provide joy and serve as an excellent outlet for stress.

Building Positive Relationships and Community

Strong social connections are vital for emotional resilience and overall well-being:

1. **Foster Relationships**:

   - Invest time in nurturing relationships with family and friends. Regular interactions and support networks can enhance feelings of belonging and security.

2. **Volunteer and Engage**:

   - Consider volunteering or participating in community activities. Getting involved can strengthen your connections with others and provide a sense of purpose.

3. **Open Communication**:

   - Practice open and honest communication with loved ones to foster healthy relationships. Sharing thoughts and feelings can strengthen bonds and resolve conflicts.

Engaging in Lifelong Learning

A commitment to lifelong learning can provide mental stimulation and keep the brain active:

1. **Pursue Educational Opportunities**:

   - Take courses, attend workshops, or participate in online learning. Subjects can range from professional development to hobbies and personal interests.

2. **Read Regularly**:

   - Reading is an accessible way to broaden knowledge and stimulate cognitive function. Explore various genres and topics to keep it engaging.

3. **Challenge Your Mind**:

   - Engage in brain-challenging activities such as puzzles, crosswords, or strategic games that promote cognitive function.

Finding Purpose and Setting Goals

A sense of purpose is essential for motivation and longevity:

1. **Identify Your Passion**:

   - Take time to reflect on what you're passionate about. Pursuing activities that align with your interests can lead to a more fulfilling life.

2. **Set Realistic Goals**:

   - Establish short- and long-term goals that provide direction and motivation. This can be related to career, health, or personal development.

3. **Celebrate Achievements**:

   - Acknowledge and celebrate your accomplishments, no matter how small. Positive reinforcement can motivate you to continue striving for your goals.

Conclusion

Making intentional lifestyle changes can significantly impact longevity and overall well-being. By prioritizing sleep, reducing stress, nurturing relationships, engaging in lifelong learning, and finding purpose, you can cultivate a vibrant and fulfilling life.

As we conclude this journey through health and well-being, remember that each small change contributes to a larger goal: a life that is not just lived longer but lived well. By embracing these principles, you can create a holistic approach to your health and well-being as you navigate the path toward a longer and healthier life. In the final section of our eBook, we will summarize the key takeaways and encourage readers to take actionable steps toward their well-being. Here's to a future filled with health, happiness, and longevity!

Chapter 8: Case Studies and Real-Life Examples

Introduction to Real-Life Stories

Understanding the principles of health and wellness is essential, but seeing how these concepts manifest in real life can be even more impactful. This chapter presents case studies and real-life examples of individuals who have made significant lifestyle changes, overcome health challenges, and adopted practices for longevity. These stories serve as inspiration and provide valuable lessons for anyone looking to enhance their health and well-being.

Case Study 1: John's Journey to Heart Health

Background: John, a 55-year-old man, was diagnosed with high blood pressure and high cholesterol. He had a sedentary lifestyle, worked long hours, and relied on fast food for his meals. Despite a family history of heart disease, John felt invincible until a routine check-up revealed alarming health measurements.

Changes Implemented:

- **Diet**: John began by educating himself about nutrition. He swapped processed foods for whole grains, fruits, and vegetables. He started meal-prepping to avoid the temptation of fast food.

- **Exercise**: John set a goal to walk 30 minutes a day. Gradually, he incorporated strength training and joined a local cycling group, which made exercise enjoyable and social.

- **Routine Check-ups**: He committed to regular check-ups with his doctor to monitor his progress.

Results: Within six months, John's blood pressure and cholesterol levels improved significantly. He lost weight, felt more energized, and reported a marked improvement in his overall mood and self-esteem. His journey highlights the importance of nutrition and physical activity in managing chronic health conditions.

Case Study 2: Maria's Mental Health Transformation

Background: Maria, a 32-year-old mother of two, struggled with anxiety and depression. After experiencing the stress of balancing family life, work, and personal challenges, Maria found herself feeling overwhelmed and isolated.

Changes Implemented:

- **Mindfulness**: Maria began practicing mindfulness and meditation for ten minutes each day, using guided meditation apps.

- **Therapy**: She sought help from a mental health professional, who provided her with coping strategies to handle stress and anxiety.

- **Support Network**: Understanding the value of community, Maria reconnected with friends and joined a local parenting group to share experiences and gain support.

Results: Over time, Maria noticed a significant reduction in her anxiety levels. Her relationships with her family and friends improved as she became more communicative and engaged. This case demonstrates the importance of seeking support and employing mindfulness techniques for mental wellness.

Case Study 3: Edward's Quest for Longevity

Background: At age 70, Edward wanted to redefine what aging meant for him. He had already faced various health challenges, including arthritis and mild diabetes. He felt that conventional wisdom dictated that he should slow down, but he sought to maintain an active and fulfilling lifestyle.

Changes Implemented:

- **Lifelong Learning**: Edward enrolled in online courses about nutrition and fitness tailored for seniors, which sparked his interest in healthy cooking.

- **Structured Exercise**: He began attending a local senior fitness class, focusing on balance, strength, and flexibility. Edward also incorporated regular walks with friends to maintain social interaction.

- **Volunteer Work**: Finding purpose was central to Edward's approach. He began volunteering at a local food pantry, which gave him a sense of contribution and fulfillment.

Results: Edward reported feeling more energetic and healthier than ever. His diabetes was better managed through dietary changes, and he gained strength and confidence from staying active. Edward's story is a testament to reimagining life in the golden years and the transformative power of purpose and community involvement.

Case Study 4: Sarah and the Power of Community

Background: Sarah, a 45-year-old woman, struggled with obesity and its associated health risks, including joint pain and low self-esteem. She felt isolated and unmotivated due to a lack of community support.

Changes Implemented:

- **Joining a Local Support Group**: Sarah found a community weight-loss group that provided encouragement, accountability, and shared experiences.

- **Nutritional Education Workshops**: She participated in nutrition workshops offered by the group, which helped her learn how to cook healthy meals and understand portion sizes.

- **Physical Activity Challenges**: Each month, the group set physical activity challenges that motivated Sarah to be more active, such as group hikes or fitness classes.

Results: After a year of commitment, Sarah lost a significant amount of weight and gained confidence. She developed lasting friendships through the support group and reported improvements in both physical and mental health. Sarah's journey emphasizes the value of community and shared experiences in achieving health goals.

Conclusion

These case studies illustrate that individuals from diverse backgrounds can adopt meaningful lifestyle changes to improve their health and well-being. Each story highlights the importance of nutrition, exercise, mental health, community support, and personal resilience in the pursuit of longevity and quality of life.

As we wrap up this chapter, remember that change is possible, and the stories of others can inspire you to embark on your journey toward a healthier future. Collectively, these examples reinforce the message that proactive health management is within reach. In the next chapter, we will summarize the key takeaways and actionable steps you can take to enhance your health and well-being, creating a roadmap toward a vibrant and fulfilling life.